# Ulcers

## *The Ultimate Cure Guide For How to Get Rid of Mouth Ulcers Instantly*

presentation of the information is without contract or any type of guarantee assurance.

The trademarks that are used are without any consent, and the publication of the trademark is without permission or backing by the trademark owner. All trademarks and brands within this book are for clarifying purposes only and are the owned by the owners themselves, not affiliated with this document.

# Table Of Contents

# Introduction

First off, I really want to thank you for downloading this book. The pages in this short e-book were developed through years of experiences that I have gone through, as well as what has proven to work for others that I have talked to and researched. I also want to congratulate you for taking the time to understand your own ulcer problems and how you can overcome them through natural techniques.

This book will cover what dietary choices you can make in order to prevent ulcers from occurring. However, for those who cannot avoid them, the remedies and treatments discussed in this book are very effective and proven to be safe. If you are one of those who are prone to getting mouth ulcers, this book is for you.

I can guarantee that you will find this useful if you make sure to implement what you learn in the following pages. The important thing is that you IMPLEMENT what you learn.

We will dive into what is going on in your mouth, how your mouth reacts to different triggers, how your eating, drinking, and hygienic habits can influence the development of ulcers, as well as what work is required of you to get past the roadblocks you have.

I recommend that you take notes while you are reading this book. This will ensure that you get the most out of the information in here. I want you to feel that you made a purchase that is worth your money and so that you can look over the notes of this book even after you've finished reading it. The notes will help you to pinpoint exactly what you need to implement, and by writing things down, you will be able to recall specifics and how to handle certain situations when they arise.

Lastly, remember that everything in this book has been compiled through research, my own experiences, as well as the experiences of others, so feel free to question what you have read in this book. I encourage you to do your own research on the things that you want to look deeper into. We must be aware of what is true and false regarding this topic, or else we become susceptible to falling for scam products like some creams and lotions that promise unrealistic results.

The more you understand about your own mind and body, the better off you'll be. To overcome mouth ulcer problems, it will take some work on your part but you can do it! So remember to read with confidence and an open mind!

# Chapter 1:

# Understanding Mouth Ulcers

A mouth ulcer, also known as a mucosal ulcer or oral ulcer, is a type of ulcer that can be found in the mucous membrane of the oral cavity. To make it simple, a mouth ulcer is an open lesion within the mouth. This type of ulcer is very common and is associated with several diseases, however, most of the time there is no serious underlying cause. The English word "ulcer" comes from the Latin word "ulcus" and from the Greek word "elkos", which mean wound.

The most common causes of mouth ulcers are local trauma and aphthous stomatitis, a condition that involves the recurrent formation of mouth ulcers for unknown reasons. An oral ulcer causes discomfort and pain and may change the individual's choice of food while the healing takes place.

# Diagnosing Mouth Ulcers

It is important to note that mouth ulcers may occur in people from any age group. They can be the result of a mild condition, such as canker sores, cold sores, gingivitis, or even from aggressive tooth brushing. In some cases, mouth ulcers can also form due to some diseases and disorders that can be serious and sometimes life-threatening. These include leukoplakia and oral cancer.

As mentioned, the formation of mouth ulcers can be due to a variety of conditions, including trauma to the gums or teeth, and as a side effect of some medications, like chemotherapy. Oral ulcers may also occur in conjunction with other symptoms which differ depending on the underlying disease, condition, or disorder. Other unusual symptoms include jaw swelling, bleeding gums, mouth pain, tooth fractures, bad breath, and unusual patches or rashes on the tongue and/or lips.

To diagnose mouth ulcers and the root causes, begin with checking the family history and medical history of the person who is dealing with them. This includes an oral X-ray and oral examination by a dentist and/or periodontist.

# Visiting Your GP or Dentist

The good news for most of you reading this e-book, is that if you only have a mild mouth ulcer, you don't need to go to your GP or personal dentist, since these ulcers will normally heal within a week or two. You need to see your GP or dentist only if you have had a very painful mouth ulcer for more than three weeks, or if you are regularly experiencing mouth ulcers off and on for over six weeks.

If you see your GP or dentist to consult, they will usually check inside your mouth to evaluate the ulcer. They may ask you some questions to determine whether your mouth ulcers have an underlying trigger or cause. For instance, you may be asked some variation of the following questions:

How often do you get mouth ulcers?

Is there someone in your family who has recurring mouth ulcers?

Are you experiencing any other symptoms such as joint pain, a rise in body temperature, or weight loss?

How long has your current ulcer lasted?

Do you smoke?

In some instances, your GP or dentist might ask you to conduct a blood test. A sample of your blood can be tested to check for any signs of inflammation or infections, as well as to check your vitamin B12 and Iron levels. Finding these levels help to determine the underlying conditions that could be responsible for your mouth ulcers.

# Chapter 2:

# Types and Common Causes of Mouth Ulcers

There are 3 main types of mouth ulcers:

Minor ulcers are the most common type, comprising of 80% of all cases. Most of the time, these are tiny in size, around two to eight millimeters in diameter. This type of ulcer heals naturally and will usually last from about ten to fourteen days. They will not lead to any scarring or any long-term damage to the mouth.

Major ulcers are bigger and deeper than minor ulcers and usually have an irregular or raised border. They are normally 1 cm or more in size. Major ulcers usually take longer to heal, normally several weeks, and may lead to long-term scarring, depending on severity.

Herpetiform ulcers form a cluster of dozens of smaller sores that are pinhead in size. The number of ulcers may range from 5 to 100. These tiny ulcers fuse together to form bigger, irregular shaped mouth sores that are very painful. Around five to ten percent of mouth ulcers are said to be herpetiform. Despite some misinformation out there, this type of ulcer is not associated with the herpes virus.

Most of the minor, single mouth ulcers are caused by damage within the mouth, for instance, by biting the wall of your cheek while eating. These ulcers will usually heal within a week or two and are not a symptom of a serious underlying problem.

# Causes of Recurrent Mouth Ulcers

The cause of recurrent mouth ulcers is not completely clear yet. However, experts are starting to believe that genes could be a big factor in recurring ulcers, mainly because it seems that around 40% of people with recurrent mouth ulcers report that it runs in their family.

# What Triggers Minor Mouth Ulcers?

Some of the factors that can trigger minor mouth ulcers are as follows:

## Anxiety and Stress

Anxiety and stress can lead people to performing odd physical behaviors, such as habitual biting of the tongue and inner wall of the mouth.

## Hormonal Changes

Some women experience mouth ulcers during their monthly period, as well as some young people (boys and girls) going through puberty.

## Eating Certain Foods

Foods like coffee, strawberries, wheat flour, chocolate, cheese, peanuts, and tomatoes can all cause ulcers within the mouth, depending on the genetics of an individual.

## Toothpaste Additives

Additives such as sodium lauryl sulphate, which is present in some toothpastes, can cause or worsen mouth ulcers in some individuals.

## Quitting Smoking

The first time a person quits smoking, they may develop mouth ulcers as they deal with the sudden change in chemical reactions within their body.

If you want to stop smoking, do not be discouraged if you develop mouth ulcers during the adjustment period. Keep in mind that the mouth ulcers are only temporary and the long-term health benefits of not smoking are infinitely better than the short-term discomfort of the ulcers.

# Medical Conditions

There are some cases wherein recurrent mouth ulcers can be a sign of an underlying medical condition, such as the following:

## Vitamin B12 Deficiency

When there is a lack of Vitamin B12 in the body, the body combats it by producing large red blood cells which cannot function properly.

## Viral Infections

Some viral infections include the cold sore virus (herpes simplex), chickenpox, and hand, foot, and mouth diseases.

## Coeliac Disease

Coeliac disease is a digestive condition where an individual has an adverse reaction to gluten.

## Iron Deficiency

Iron deficiency is when a lack of iron in the bloodstream results in the reduction of the amount of oxygen reaching a person's tissues and organs.

## Chron's Disease

Chron's disease is a long-term condition that causes inflammation in the lining of the digestive system.

## Behcet's Disease

Behcet's disease is a rare condition that causes inflammation of the blood vessels.

## Reactive Arthritis

Reactive arthritis is a condition that causes inflammation in different areas of the body, usually due to infection.

## Lichen Planus

Lichen Planus is a non-infectious, itchy rash that can harm many parts of the body.

## Immunodeficiency

Immunodeficiency is when the immune system of the body is attacked or suppressed, for instance, in Lupus or HIV.

Bullous pemphigoid is a rare type of skin disease which features tense blistering eruptions on the skin's surface. This condition is caused by the antibodies and inflammation accumulating in a specific layer of the skin and mucous membranes.

Cancer sores, or aphthous stomatitis, are tiny, painful ulcers in the mouth. The sores may occur on the tongue or on the lining of the lips, throat, and cheeks. They are white, yellow, or gray in color with a red border.

Dry mouth is a condition that normally leads to the reduced production of saliva. With this condition, a person will experience difficulties speaking and may suffer from mal-nutrition. Extreme dry mouth and salivary gland dysfunction may result in permanent throat and mouth disorders that can impair the person's quality of life. Xerostomia is another name for dry mouth.

Gingivitis, or gum disease, is the inflammation of the tissues supporting and surrounding the teeth, which is caused by poor dental hygiene. Gingivitis is a very common condition and differs widely in severity. One symptom includes red, swollen gums that bleed easily when brushing the teeth. Gingivitis and periodontitis are not the same, although there are instances in which a person may acquire both.

Herpangina is a self-limited, acute, virally induced illness often occuring in young children during the summer months. Affected children normally complain of fever and mouth sores. Herpangina is caused by several viruses, all belonging to the enterovirus family, coxsackievirus being the most popular.

Most children who develop a high fever and sore throat will have ulcers develop at the back of the palate and throat. Children, particularly younger children, may not want to eat or drink because of the pain they feel, and are at risk of having signs and symptoms of dehydration.

Leukoplakia is characterized by the presence of white or gray colored patches on the gums, the inside of the cheeks, tongue, and/or roof of the mouth. The patches may develop slowly over weeks to months, and are thick, slightly raised, and may take on a rough and hardened texture. They are painless most of the time, but sensitive to touch, spicy foods, heat, or other irritations.

Thrush is the medical condition in which fungus, known as Candida albicans, overgrow in the throat and mouth. This can be caused by a variety of factors, including medications, dentures, smoking, pregnancy, and other illnesses.

# Treatments That May Cause Mouth Ulcers

Most chemotherapy drugs can cause mouth sores, but this adverse effect is more frequent with some other treatments. Below is a list of chemotherapy drugs that have been known to cause mouth ulcers in roughly 30% or more of the patients who consume them:

Trimetrexate (Neutrexin®, TMQ®, TMTX®)

Tretinoin (Vesanoid®)

Teniposide (Vumon®)

Procarbazine (Matulane®)

Plicamycin (Mithracin®)

Pemetrexed (Alimta®)

Paclitaxel (Taxol®, Onxal™)

Oprevelkin (Neumega®)

Mitoxantrone (Novantrone®)

Mitomycin (Mutamycin®)

Methotrexate (Rheumatrex®, Trexall™)

Mechlorethamine (Mustargen®)

Liposomal doxorubicin (Doxil®)

Isotretinoin (Accutane®)

Idarubicin (Idamycin®, Idamycin PFS®)

Fluorouracil (5-FU, Adrucil®, Carac®, Efudex®, Fluoroplex®)

Floxuridine (FUDR®)

Epirubicin (Ellence®)

Doxorubicin (Adriamycin®, Rubex®)

Docetaxel (Taxotere®)

Daunorubicin (Cerubidine®)

Cytarabine (Cytosar-U®)

Busulfan (Myleran®, Busulfex®)

Actinomycin (Cosmegen)

Here is a list of chemotherapy drugs that have been known to cause mouth ulcers in about 10-29% of patients:

Vincristine (Oncovin®, Vincasar PFS®)

Vinblastine (Velban®, Alkaban AQ®)

Tretinoin (Vesanoid®)

Trastuzumab (Herceptin®)

Topotecan (Hycamtin®)

Thiotepa (Thioplex®)

Rasburicase (Elitek®)

Pentostatin (Nipent®)

Oxaliplatin (Eloxatin®)

Melphalan (Alkeran®)

Lomustine (CeeNU®)

Liposomal daunorubicin (DaunoXome®)

Irinotecan (Camptosar®)

Interleukin 2 (Proleukin®)

Hydroxyurea (Hydrea®)

Gemtuzumab ozogamicin (Mylotarg®)

Gemcitabine (Gemzar®)

Etoposide (VePesid®, Toposar®, Etopophos®)

Cyclophosphamide (Cytoxan®, Neosar®)

Carboplatin (Paraplatin®)

Capecitabine (Xeloda®)

Bleomycin (Blenoxane®)

Asparaginase (Elspar®, Kidrolase®)

Alemtuzumab (Campath®)

Also, mouth ulcers can occur in other forms of treatment for cancer. Mouth ulcers are even more severe if you are being treated with the following:

Combined chemotherapy and radiation therapy

Frequent dosing schedules, such as weekly chemotherapy

High-dose treatment

Radiation for head and neck cancer

Stem cell transplants

Some techniques in administering radiation may also affect the severity and duration of mouth ulcers. The following radiation techniques may produce less severe side effects:

IMRT, or Intensify Modulated Radiation Therapy, spares normal tissues, reducing mouth ulcers, while still providing the full radiation dose, or even an increased dose to the cancer.

Hyper-fractionated radiation involves lower doses taken more frequently, which result in less severe adverse effects.

# Chapter 3:

# How to Prevent Mouth Ulcers via Proper Diet

Some great news is that the connection between mouth ulcers and diet is well-established. There are certain dietary habits, like eating acidic or other irritating foods, that can cause mouth ulcers, while other eating habits may help to prevent the occurrence of mouth ulcers. Here are five helpful dietary tips that can help prevent ulcers from occurring inside your mouth.

# Increase Your Vitamin B12 and Vitamin B9 Intake

Cobalamin, or Vitamin B12, has been known to be very effective at treating mouth ulcers. A study was conducted, where 58 people with mouth ulcers were given a dose of 1,000 mcg of Vitamin B12. The duration of the outbreaks, number of ulcers, and the level of pain linked to the mouth ulcers, decreased greatly after five months of taking Vitamin B12. Also, 74% of patients in this group reported no mouth ulcers at the end of the study.

Likewise, Vitamin B9, also known as folic acid, has properties that may help prevent mouth ulcers, especially in individuals who are deficient in this essential vitamin.

# Reduce Alcohol Intake

Another helpful diet tip for preventing the occurrence of mouth ulcers is to reduce alcohol consumption. Consuming too much alcohol can deplete the stores of Vitamin B, including Vitamin B12 and Vitamin B9.

# Eat Foods Rich in Iron

An iron deficiency is the most common form of nutritional deficiency in Western countries and it has been linked to recurrent mouth ulcers. Women who are having their periods, women who are anticipating or have just given birth, long-distance runners, as well as vegans, have a particularly high risk of becoming deficient in iron.

Start including more iron-rich foods into your diet, such as fruits, liver, oysters, egg yolks, salmon, tuna, lean red meat, spinach, poultry, and whole grains. It should also be noted that your doctor can check your blood levels to determine if you have any nutritional deficiencies and can help you to supplement your diet accordingly.

# Eliminate Food Allergens

Mouth ulcers can also be caused by food allergens and intolerances, and thus getting rid of food allergens may be the ideal dietary tip for individuals who suffer from recurrent mouth ulcers. It is essential to remember, however, that what causes an allergic reaction in one individual may not trigger the same reaction in another. Some of the most common food allergens include soy products, wheat, dairy, eggs, and yeast.

Other popular allergens that people with mouth ulcers may be sensitive to, are certain preservatives and food additives like tartrazine, monosodium glutamate, sulfites, and benzoates. Benzoates are anti-microbial preservatives that are used in soft drinks as well as some food items. Tartrazine is one of the most commonly used artificial food colorings, and it is present in several processed foods in different proportions.

Items that may contain tartrazine are usually orange or yellow colored soft drinks, candy, instant soups, pasta brands, chips, confectionery, canned vegetables, pickled products, cereals, butter, and some cheeses. MSG, or Monosodium glutamate, is a flavor enhancer used in several processed foods as well as in foods cooked in Chinese restaurants.

Sulfites are usually added to alcoholic beverages and dried fruits in order to lengthen their shelf life. The perfect way to ensure your "anti-mouth ulcers diet" is free of preservatives and additives is to choose natural, organic foods that have undergone minimal chemical additives and processing.

You can also carry out an allergy test at an allergy clinic to determine whether you are allergic to certain substances in your diet. The best way to go about knowing potential allergens is to complete an elimination diet under the supervision of a nutritionist. This diet includes removing foods and substances that are suspected of causing allergic reactions for several weeks.

If after the period of elimination, symptoms have improved or cleared significantly, the suspected substances and foods can be re-introduced slowly. At this stage, the dieter methodically goes through all the suspected allergens, one by one, by taking a suspected substance or food many times a day and then returning to the elimination diet for a few days.

If the symptoms re-occur or get worse during those days, the dieter could be allergic to the chemical or food that was re-introduced. Even though the elimination diet is fairly simple to complete, the entire process can take up to several months and does require patience and discipline.

# Avoid Spicy and Acidic Foods

If you are prone to getting mouth ulcers, you will benefit from avoiding spicy or acidic foods. These foods may irritate your mouth, which can lead to the development of mouth ulcers. Examples include sour candies, such as Warheads or Sour Patch Kids, as well as very spicy peppers and sauces.

# Chapter 4:

# Ways to Get Rid of Mouth Ulcers

Minor mouth ulcers usually last from around four to fourteen days, however, treatment can help to protect the ulcer from further damage, numb the pain, and decrease the possibilities of bacterial infection. Some medications may speed up the healing if used at an early stage. Here are some medications that you can use in treating mouth ulcers:

### Aloclair Gel

This is an aloe vera extract with hyaluronic acid and it can help to stop mouth ulcers from worsening.

## Orlamedic

This is a medicated lotion that can be applied to the mouth ulcers using cotton buds to create a seal over the ulcer.

## Forever Bright Toothgel

This can be utilized when brushing or it can be applied to the ulcers directly. This can be especially helpful if your current toothpaste causes irritation to the ulcers when brushing.

## Weleda Medicinal Gargle

This is a combination of several essential oils that will help in getting rid of pain due to the anti-bacterial properties that it consists of.

## Iglu Gel

This creates a protective covering over the ulcers which help to get rid of infection and reduce pain in the area.

# Products Used in Coating and Healing the Ulcers

## Over the Counter Products

The common remedies that you can purchase over the counter can form a long lasting layer of protection over the ulcers. These products are available in the form of gels as well as liquid paints. They contain anti-inflammatory ingredients and may prevent the ulcers from getting worse, if used during the early development period. Make sure to dry the ulcers using a cotton bud before applying any products.

You can ask your pharmacist for assistance in choosing the most appropriate treatment for your mouth ulcer. Apply gels and pastes during the day. You can also apply at bedtime to enable longer contact with the mouth sores. If the pain is too much, you can also take a pain reliever such as paracetamol. If you are pregnant or breastfeeding, check with your pharmacist and doctor before using any products.

## Paste Treatments

The pastes form a protective covering over the ulcer, which help the medicine adhere to the ulcer. This makes the healing process faster and can lessen the pain. Some pastes have anti-inflammatory properties that, if applied during the tingling stage, can stop the mouth ulcer from developing even further.

You may be required to dry your mouth first before applying the paste. Remember to dab it instead of rubbing it in.

## Gel Treatments

Some gels can numb the pain upon forming a protective layer over the ulcer. Avoid applying large amounts of gels, particularly in children under twelve years of age. Over the counter gels will have recommendations regarding the amount and frequency to apply.

## Liquid Paint Treatments

Liquid paint treatments create a protective layer over the ulcers but also need to be re-applied often. If you are willing to apply it multiple times a day, this could be the option for you.

## Mouthwash

Mouthwash is helpful for hard to reach mouth ulcers as well as when there are numerous ulcers in the mouth at the same time. They can help to prevent bacteria from causing an infection and some can even help numb the pain as well.

It is best if you start using the product as soon as there is a tingling sensation in a developing ulcer.

## Liquorice

A type of liquorice known as DGL, or deglycrhizinated liquorice, can be used to cover mouth ulcers. You can purchase it in the form of small wafers from some health food shops. You can chew one or two wafers around two to three times a day for optimal effects.

## Aloe Vera

As mentioned earlier, Aloe Vera sap can help numb the pain created by mouth ulcers. If possible, squeeze some sap out from the plant itself. Dry the mouth ulcer using a cotton bud and then dab onto the sap. The great thing is that you can do this as often as you'd like.

## Vitamin E

Vitamin E oil is also very helpful in this process. Cut a vitamin E capsule in half and squeeze some on the affected area.

## Dump Tea Bags

Dump tea bags are alkaline and have astringent properties. Putting one on the affected area for 5 minutes will help to neutralize the acid and lessen overall pain in the mouth.

## Topical Anesthetics

Topical anesthetics such as Rinstead gel or Anbesol liquid can be re-applied several times a day.

## Hydrogen Peroxide

Hydrogen peroxide is a powerful disinfectant. Combine hydrogen peroxide with half a glass of water. Put one tablespoon of bicarbonate soda and one teaspoon of salt, then stir until all the substances appear to be dissolved. Swish the solution around in your mouth and spit it out after 30 seconds to a minute.

## Calendula

Calendula is commonly known as garden marigold, which has been used for many years in treating minor cuts, insect bites, and cracked skin conditions. Pour boiling water into a cup, add two teaspoons of dried marigold petals, and allow it to cool down. Gargle and swish the tea around in your mouth as frequently as you want.

## Vitamin C

Vitamin C with flavonoids will aid in healing the mucous membrane of the mouth. Daily intake of Vitamin C can also help tremendously in reducing the occurrence of mouth ulcers by preventing them from forming.

## Propolis from the Beehive

Before using other natural remedies, many experts recommend that you try Propolis first. A drop of Propolis directly on the ulcerated area a few times a day can heal the mouth ulcers quickly. It will produce a sharp sensation for a second or two but the pain does not last long. If you can not find Propolis, you can try the Calendula, as mentioned above.

## Coconut Oil

Coconut oil has been known as a great home remedy for many diseases, including mouth ulcers. It was used in primitive societies for many years as one of the primary healing tools. Studies have shown that it can kill certain types of bacteria altogether, which makes it one of the best remedies for mouth ulcers. Just rub the oil directly onto the affected areas twice a day and you will notice a great difference.

## Turmeric Powder

Combine a pinch amount of turmeric powder to one teaspoon of glycerine and apply it on the affected area. This is one of the simplest home remedies for mouth sores.

## Indian Gooseberry

Create a paste of amia, or Indian Gooseberry, and then apply it to the affected area two to three times a day.

## Basil Leaves

Chew on five to six tulsi, or basil leaves, and drink some water along with it. Repeat this five to six times a day if you are getting positive results from the first few experiences.

## Aciclovir

Aciclovir is an anti-viral medication that may help in treating mouth ulcers due to the herpes simplex virus. It should be applied when there is a tingling, not painful, sensation in the mouth.

Ayurvedic Medicine can relieve the pain of mouth ulcers. Ayurvedic is an Indian system that believes ulcers and sores come from the symptoms of high pitta. This type of medication treats mouth ulcers using a pitta-soothing diet that avoids spicy and hot foods and recommends cranberry juice in-between meals, in order to relieve pain and inflammation. An aloe vera gel is applied three times per day and you can use aloe vera juice as mouthwash to ease the pain and inflammation.

Treating the underlying cause of mouth sores, or ulcers, is a significant step, however, you can use several remedies to relieve pain and inflammation. The condition may or may not respond to medication right away, but you will be able to tell which ones are helping after just a couple of hours.

# Chapter 5:

# Additional Types of Mouth Ulcers

There are several types of mouth ulcers that seldomly occur, two of which are as follows:

## Angular Chelitis

This type of mouth ulcer is caused by a fungus known as candida albicans, which is responsible for several intra-oral fungal infections. It is characterized by cracked fissures found at the corners of the mouth and tender tissues surrounded by flaky skin. This type of mouth ulcer can be mild to very painful, depending on how severe it is.

Angular Chelitis is triggered by deep folds at the edges of the mouth, often due to dentures, bite collapse, and other predisposed infections. This type of mouth ulcer occurs due to weather, trauma, habits, and the like. Reduced oral immunity due to diabetes, HIV, illness, medications, diabetes, and others, can make a person susceptible to oral fungal infections.

It is actually worsened by patients licking their lips trying to soothe the symptoms, because it adds more fungus to the lesions. It is treated using anti-inflammatory/anti-fungal ointments and may disappear after a few days.

# Lichen Planus

Lichen Planus is a benign dermatologic condition that occurs within the mouth; however, there is no apparent skin involvement. It can occur if the person has a weak immune system and can be caused by specific medications.

Lichen Planus is characterized by a lacy, white pattern of different sizes and may occur anywhere within the mouth, though the inner cheek is the most common place of occurrence. This type of mouth ulcer is asymptomatic and sometimes patients are not aware they actually have it, unless their dentist notifies them. The lesion ranges in size, from near remission to full mouth involvement.

This type of mouth ulcer is quite painful. The ulcerated part can also become very big and bothersome and will last several weeks sans treatment. There are no apparent triggers outside of stress, poor nutrition, and galvanic reactions to fillings. It can be treated by applying topical steroids. Needless to say, stress reduction and good nutrition can also help to reduce the occurrence of ulcerative episodes.

# Conclusion

Thank you again for downloading this book!

I worked hard on creating the best guide for "overcoming mouth ulcers" that I could. These are all the strategies and information that has worked for me, as well as others that I have talked to and researched. I guarantee if you stay consistent they will work for you as well. Be optimistic about your current situation and make small progress each day!

If you feel like you learned something from this book, please take the time to share your thoughts with me by sending me a message. I would also appreciate it if you left a review on Amazon, as I love hearing back from those who have tried out these methods. It would be greatly appreciated!

Thank you and good luck in your journey!